REGENERATIVE FOODS BLOOD GROUP AB DIABETIC

ISBN 978-1-312-26047-4

www.fundaciondeterapeutas.com

MANUEL RAMONI... NEURO-THERAPIST

Worse Foods (Blood Bundles, Sick and Aged). ___Wheat, Corn, Pork, Chicken, Delicatessen, Avocado, Tomato, Fried Meals, Shrimp, Peanuts, White Sugar___

FOOD ACCORDING TO YOUR BLOOD GROUP.

BLOOD GROUP "AB DIABETIC" - THE ENIGMA.

What you will learn in the following pages will change your life and that of your loved ones forever and in such a precise and safe way that in a few weeks they will feel the changes in their body in such a radical and different way, that They will feel and will be younger, stronger, more vigorous, full of energy, vitality and most importantly ... Full of great **health and that when any viral or bacterial disease wants to enter their body, they will hardly feel a breakdown since** their immune system and **"ALKALINITY"** (I will teach you later) - it will be so strong that it will be almost impossible for them to ever get sick again (this if they keep their new culture of feeding and living that I will teach them for life) and therefore lead them to live the average 100-year-old.

Dr. Peter D`adamo, a deeply scientific researcher and pioneer in the field of food according to blood groups, has managed to compile through many scientific studies in different cultures and around many countries in the world. The way and way of classifying food according to the type of blood of human beings.

He managed to bring as much food as possible to the laboratory on his tour around the world and took each food and looked at it through the microscope with a blood sample of the different types that there are (4), type "O" - "A" - "B" and "AB" and managed to observe very carefully what was happening.

He managed to see that by placing the different types of food in the different types of blood, that these presented totally different characteristics from each other, that is; A) That there was a group of foods that made the blood more fluid, light and thin. B) A second group made absolutely no changes to it. C) While a third group surprisingly had clumping of the blood, that is, it made it thick and even coagulated.

So I manage to divide the food very intelligently and amazingly into three groups.

1- The foods that make the blood more fluid and less viscous or thick, making it feed (Carrying oxygen) in a very important way to all the cells of the body, passing through the thinnest capillaries of the body, nourishing, regenerating them and rejuvenating cell tissue in an extremely vital way for the body. As well as at the same time making the minute volume of the heart the most suitable for the body, thus reducing the overload that the heart needs when the blood is thick and very intoxicated... And he called them **VERY BENEFICIAL FOODS.**

2-   A second group of foods that did not present or give any change in blood behavior that called them **NEUTRAL FOODS.**

3-   And a third group of foods in which he noticed that in a very important way they presented clumping of the blood, making it more viscous and thick and thus hindering its function to the point that it was the main cause of premature cellular aging and called: **HARMFUL FOODS, NOT ADVISABLE OR "POISON" FOOD.** Therefore it determined after deep studies that each blood group has its indispensable food pattern and different from each other, that is, the foods that can be beneficial for a certain blood group... It is totally harmful to others.

1) **VERY   BENEFICIAL:** Rejuvenate, Slim, Regenerate, Regulate Cardiac Minute Volume And Extend Life.

2) **NEUTRAL: They** feed but do not regenerate, nor do anything that group 1 does.

3) **NOT ADVISABLE:** They fatten, agglutinate (Thicken) the blood, poison the body, overload the heart, age and degenerate the cellular system.

Below I am going to expose you after many years of study and research on my part, as I have managed to summarize in broad terms the foods according to each blood group.

This I achieved thanks to GOD in tens of thousands of patients that I have seen in more than 39 years of consultation and follow-up, which with a lot of work and diligence I carried out in the deep study of each food in each blood group. Therefore, each region, country and its customs are of utmost importance.

For example, in the case of Venezuela there is the custom of the so-called pre-cooked flour or "bread flour", which has been consumed in large proportions in Venezuelan households for more than 66 years, and I realized that the sub generations following the continuous consumption of certain foods that are in principle of the group of harmful, the body adapts to the same for living and converts food HARMFUL food NEUTROS, with low toxicity, depending on the degree of generations that have crossed.

Other examples would be: Mexico, Chile (Spicy), Panamá, The Fritters, Brazil, La Feijoada (Black beans), Colombia the potatoes, Spain, Wine, etc.

Another thing that I learned unequivocally through so many years of monitoring, practice and study, is that; There are industrialized "foods" on the market that they sell to consumers in order to lose weight by substituting some of the main meals for a shake, which among other things, poorly combining, refined and industrialized carbohydrates with processed proteins (highly harmful combination, (Which we will talk about on the alkalinity life - acidification and death) In the Complete Guide to Healthy Longevity ...

That it "loses weight" but "dries" them at the same time, since the loss of collagen is progressive, and worst of all is that after the patient having spent fortunes on these "foods" they gain weight again unless they follow the diet regimen. "Products", something that will never happen with The Aliments According to its Blood Group.

There are basically three different types of protein shakes depending on the source from which those proteins are obtained, which may well be from whey (Poison for group O), egg white or soy (Poison for other groups) . The consumer does not have the slightest idea of how their body is poisoned (Acidifying it) with these drinks that keep them "full" but that far from nourishing the immune system, what is sinking it in an ending that always ends up leading to the query.

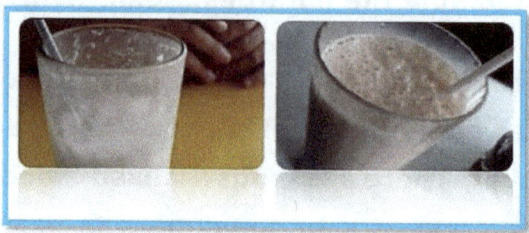

Scientific researchers at the University of California, San Francisco studied 9,000 women and found that those who consumed these products were about four times more likely to have hip fractures, among other things, than those who did not consume these "foods."

An unbalanced diet (Since it is the same "food" for everyone equally... "And no one is the same as another", especially in your blood group) "high in proteins, such as those from shakes, will directly contribute to having fragile bones or osteoporosis among other serious conditions that you will have in the medium or short term, more likely in some than others, depending on your vitality and blood group.

"Eating these artificial and highly harmful" foods "is like smoking and saying ... "It doesn't hurt me"

Keep in mind that according to the different food cultures that I will indicate for each blood group in particular, there are also people who are "secretory" and "non-secretory".

SECRETORS. A person is secretory, regardless of their blood group. It is when the antigens of your blood group are present both in your blood and in your body fluids and secretions, such as saliva, intestinal mucus or respiratory cavities, semen, etc.

NO SECRETARIES. A non-secretor, it does not secrete antigen from its group in its fluids but only in its blood.

Many metabolic characteristics such as carbohydrate intolerance or immune susceptibilities are genetically linked to the non-secretory subtype. A certain disadvantage is supposed compared to the "secretors", since these, when secreting the antigen from their blood group in their saliva and the intestinal mucus, have "extra" protection against certain microorganisms and lectins of some foods.

Another additional advantage of secretors is that they are able to maintain a more stable ecosystem of bifid intestinal bacteria suitable for their group. Most of these bifid bacteria use their blood group as the preferred food source, and since secretors have a higher blood volume in the intestinal mucus, their bacteria benefit from a more constant supply of food.

Approximately 80% of the world population are "secretaries". While 20% are Non-Secretaries. Therefore, it is important to repeat that the following list of foods according to your blood group has been adapted to correct these disagreements when shopping at the supermarket. And something of which I will be very emphatic... DO NOT PUT ANY FOOD OUT OF YOUR BLOOD GROUP IN THE CART WHEN MAKING THE MARKET for you.

With this new culture of eating, you will be able to eat whatever you want and as many times as you want to eat, as long as it is in the range of foods indicated according to your blood group, such as those that are advisable and neutral, but never the "poisons". You will not only lose weight quickly and progressively, but a date will come when you will not lose weight anymore since at that moment you will have reached your ideal natural weight and can continue eating as many times as you want during the day and **NOT** You will never gain more weight in your life and if you are a thin person, then not only will you feel better, but you will soon be in your necessary size and according to your age, but with a full immune system on top and prepared to fight any attack exogenous...

It is for this and other reasons that you will see in the course of the content of this Guide that I have successfully managed to eradicate diseases from a sick body and cure patients ranging from simple obesity to cancer of any kind and thanks to *GOD*. In more than 45 years of experience and unless it is due to natural causes, I HAVE NEVER LOST A PATIENT...

BLOOD TYPE "AB DIABETIC" - THE ENIGMA

It is the modern fusion of groups A and B. It has the chameleon's response to changing food and environmental conditions, a sensitive digestive tract, an overly tolerant immune system. Spiritually, he responds better to stress, with physical vigor and creative energy and with calm action.

It is a mystery of evolution. Only 2% to 5% of the world population have this type of blood. **ABs like to say emotionally that they carry the same blood of Jesus Christ in their body, since according to the tests carried out on the Shroud of Turin, the Son of GOD possessed the type of blood AB.**

They have a spiritual and slightly sparkling personality, which makes them very attractive and popular. They welcome us with open arms, they don't hold a grudge when we snub them, and they always say things diplomatically. **Your natural charisma can often lead to heartbreak** (suffering, grief, sadness, anguish, anxiety, and intense worry caused by danger or threat).

Multiple antigens sometimes make it look like A or B and sometimes a fusion of the two, which can be positive or negative depending on the circumstances.

It shares with type A the susceptibility to breast cancer. If you have a family history, incorporate **snails (Helix Pomatia)** into your diet, as it contains a powerful lectin that binds together the mutant cells of two of the most common forms of breast cancer.

Basically, foods that are contraindicated for groups A and B are for AB, but there are exceptions.

The panhemoaglutinantes are better tolerated and those of **the type AB can eat tomatoes without problems.**

You gain weight if you eat unwise meats, which you can replace with vegetables and tofu (soy cheese). Inhibited insulin production causes hypoglycemia and a drop in blood sugar after meals, leading to less efficient metabolism of food.

Group AB does not have a severe reaction to wheat gluten but you should avoid it because it increases **the acid in your muscle tissue** and this type uses calories better when your tissue is more alkaline.

People who want to lose weight and volume or are diabetic, necessarily have to suspend, sweets, beer, flour and carbohydrates during weight loss treatment either Very Beneficial or Neutrals. Because they interfere with the purification of the body. And after they have finished and are at their ideal weight they can eat these foods as long as they are in the allowed foods.

The "AB Diabetic"
Group tolerates quite well

Cereals and Dairy.

- **Red meat:** Poorly digested, they are stored as fat.

- **Beans:** They inhibit insulin efficiency and cause hypoglycemia.

- **Beans-beans:** Inhibit insulin efficiency, cause hypoglycemia.

- **Sesame seeds:** They cause hypoglycemia:

- **Wheat:** Slows metabolism inefficient use of calories and also inhibits insulin efficiency.

- It is the least frequent of all 4% of Caucasians and blacks carry it.

- It is the most recently developed blood type.

- They are able to digest and assimilate without problems almost all foods allowed, provided they are in good condition.

- Regarding their tendencies, they meet both the inclinations of those in group "A" and those of group "B".

- According to some scientists, people who carry this "AB" blood group have great spiritual sensitivity.

Next I will indicate the list of foods for group AB DIABETIC updated and compiled with studies of many years of strategic follow-up for each blood group. These will make them lose overweight and diseases of any kind of which they are possessors with knowledge or that these diseases are in full development and you do not know it yet.

PEOPLE WHO WANT TO LOWER THEIR WEIGHT AND VOLUME.

They have to suspend, the **sweets, beers, flours and all carbohydrates** during the treatment to lose weight, whether they are Very **Beneficial** or Neutral. Because they interfere with the purification of the body. And after they have reached their ideal weight they will be able to eat these foods as long as they are in the beneficial foods.

Next I will indicate the list of foods for group A updated and compiled with studies of many years of strategic follow-up for each blood group. That will make them lose overweight and diseases of any kind of which they are possessors with knowledge or that these diseases are in full development and you do not know it yet.

It is of utmost importance due to the change of name of foods according to the region, the country or the culture; that when they get the name of a food in the lists that I indicate below and they do not know it. **Search the Internet with the name of the food and its**

synonym. Then with **the name of the food in question, look** in the part of **Google images** and thus you can recognize the food.

FORMULA FOR THE "AB DIABETIC" GROUP.

It is very important to eat the three main meals and the three snacks since your metabolism without the constant consumption of food due to your intellectual need for energetic-cerebral work ... You should never miss your snacks (in addition to what you want to eat within your meals allowed) fruits, vegetable salads with salmon and cereals.

MEATS ALLOWED	10%
FISH AND SEAFOOD	25%
BIRDS AND EGGS	5 %
BENEFICAL VEGETABLES	40%
FRUITS	15 %
CEREALS AND GRAINS	5 %

Practice this formula the best you can and you will see in a short time how it reduces your disease until it disappears completely from your body in cases of type 2 and type 3 diabetes. While in type 1 diabetes or insulin dependent mellitus you will gradually notice how their diabetes is reduced until in many cases the habit of taking insulin is eliminated, in others until the dependence on insulin is drastically reduced. While in the most chronic cases it will reduce at least between 40 and 60% of

insulin dependence, achieving in all cases profoundly improving the person's quality of life.

In diabetic groups, it is practically the same formula as non-diabetic groups. The difference is that the diabetic groups have to eliminate their sugar and excess carbohydrates to bring them to a safe cure in cases of type 2 and 3 diabetes, while in cases of type 1 diabetes or insulin-dependent in many cases insulin it will be eliminated by installing the new culture that I present to you in this Guide, (But above all in the indications and recommendations that you will find in the Healthy Longevity Guide) and in other cases not only will the amount of insulin that is injected daily be considerably reduced, but also it will greatly improve your quality of life.

MEATS AND BIRDS.

Girls should eat portions and spaced **choosing lamb, mutton, rabbit and turkey** instead of **beef**.

Avoid smoked and cured meats that can cause stomach cancer in people with low levels of gastric acid.

Very Beneficial: Ram (sheep, sheep), Lamb (lamb, goat, goat), Rabbit, Turkey.

Neutral: Ostrich, Pheasant.

Not Recommended: Squirrel, Buffalo, Beef, Horse, Goat, Pork, Quail, Heart, Cornish Chicken, Delicatessen or Fried Food, Goose, Pigeon, Duck,

Partridge, Chicken, Veal (beef), Bacon, Turtle, Venison.

FISH AND SEAFOOD.

They are an excellent source of protein for group AB. **If susceptible to breast cancer, eat Helix Pomatia snails.**

Very Beneficial: Tuna, Cod, Sea Bream, Mackerel (bonito), Snail Helix pomatia (it is the only snail that this group should eat, without exception), Dolphin, Sturgeon, Horse Mackerel, Grouper, Meeerbrasse, Oceanic Perch, Red Snapper, White Snapper , Monkfish, Sailfish, Monkfish, Shad, Salmon, Sardine.

Neutrals : Abalone (abalone), Anjova, Fresh Herring, Catfish, Squid, Carp, Carite, Catalan, Cataco, Caviar, Dogfish, Corocoro, Corégono, Corbina, Cubera, Dorado, Smelt, Lisa (Lebranche, Pataruca, Múgil) , Lofolátilo (sweet potato fish in Brazil), Pike, Mussels, Palometa (pompano), Rio Perch, Swordfish, Moonfish, Parrotfish, Salpa, Shark, Trilla (mullet in Spain), Scallops.

Not Recommended: Haddock, Clam, Anchovy, Eel, Frog's Leg, Pickled Herring, Blue Whiting, Barracuda, Beluga, Lobster, Brosmio, Shrimp, Crab, Snails (Helix Pomatia Si) , White Sturgeon, Haddock, Prawns, Salmon Eggs, Halibut, Lobster, Prawns, Gray Sole, Medregal, Hake, Mollusks, Oysters, Deep Frozen Fish, Flounder, Octopus, Frog, Snook, Turbot, Smoked Salmon, Rainbow Trout, Sea Trout, Turtle.

DAIRY AND EGGS.

Control mucus (sinusitis, ear infections, and respiratory conditions) that indicate the need to reduce dairy, especially fermented and cultured skim. Use two egg whites for each yolk to lower cholesterol. **The lectin present in chicken muscle tissue is not in the egg.**

Very Beneficial: Skim Sour Cream, Cottage, Kefir, Goat Milk, Mozzarella, Goat Cheese, Sheep Cheese (feta) , Ranchero Cheese (Farmerkäse), Ricotta Cheese, Yogurt.

Neutrals: Casein, Curd, Soy Cream, Gruyere, Gouda, Jarlsburg, Eggs 3 to 4 weekly (goose, chicken, quail), Almond Milk, Soy Milk (little), Skim Cow's Milk, Munsters, Neufchatel, Cheese Ball (Edamer), Colby Cheese, Cheddar Cheese (little), Melted Cheese, Gruyere Cheese, Fresh Cheese, Hüttenkäse Cheese , Peanut Margarine, Walnut Margarine, Whey, Swiss, Whey.

Not Recommended: Camembert, Emmenthal, Ice Cream (with cow's milk), Duck Eggs, Cut Milk, Whole Milk, Coconut Milk, Butter, Butter (animal), Brie Cheese, Blue Cheese, Camembert Cheese, Brie Cheese, Emmentaler Cheese, Parmesan, Provolone, Roquefort, Sorbet.

OILS AND FATS.

Use olive oil instead of animal fats, hydrogenated vegetables or other vegetable oils.

Very Beneficial: Olive Oil, Walnut Oil.

Neutrals: Coconut Oil (little), Wheat Germ Oil, Soybean Oil, Blackcurrant Oil, Rapeseed Oil, Almond Oil, Evening Primrose Oil, Castor Oil, Borage Oil, Cod liver oil, Linseed Oil, Peanut Oil.

Not Recommended: Canola Oil, Safflower Oil, Sunflower Oil, Corn Oil, Cotton Oil, Sesame Oil.

DRIED FRUITS AND SEEDS.

In small amounts and with caution because they contain insulin inhibitory lectins and can affect your gallbladder.

Very Beneficial: Chestnuts, Peanuts, Peanut Butter.

Neutral: Almond, Cocoa, Mushrooms, Beech, Dried Figs without sugar, Dried Apricots without sugar, Almond Margarine, Merey, Nefelio, Walnut, Pecan, Pine nuts, Pistachio, Safflower Seeds, Linseed Seeds.

Not Recommended: Hazelnut, Butter or Sunflower Margarine, Butter or Sesame Margarine, Sesame Seeds, Poppy Seeds, Pumpkin Seeds.

VEGETABLES.

Lentils are a very important food to fight cancer in type AB due to their antioxidants. But the grains should be eaten in small quantities until their diabetic greed is eliminated.

Very Beneficial: Soy Beans, Pinto Beans, Green Lentils (peas).

Neutral: Coffee in Beans (little), Broad Bean, White Bean, Beans (little), Soy Beans, Red Lentils, Soy Products, Jicama Bean, Tofu (soy cheese), Pods.

Not Recommended: Beans, Caraota, Red Beans, Chickpeas, Green Bean.

CEREALS. (Very little).

If you have asthma or are overweight, avoid wheat. Limit germ and wheat bran to once a week.

Very Beneficial: Oats, Amaranth, Puffed Rice, Rice Crackers, Brown Rice, Basmati Rice, Rice-based Drink (rice chicha, bottle, atoll), Cream and Rice Flour, Spelled, Millet, Oat Bran, Bran Rice, Brown Rice. "DIABETIC" people should suspend these foods until they are free of diabetes.

Neutral: Barley, Rye or Rye Flour, Starch, Wheat Germ, Granola, Soy Granules, Soy Flakes, Malt, Quinoa, Wheat Bran (bran), Wheat Semolina (pasta), Crumbled Wheat. "DIABETIC" people should suspend these foods until they are free of diabetes.

Not Recommended: White Rice, Sesame, Pop Corn, Casabe, White or Yellow Corn Flour, Jojoto or Elote,

Cassava Flour, Corn Flakes, Kasha, Corn of No Kind, Sorghum Millet, Buckwheat.

BREADS. (Very little)

If you produce excessive mucus or are overweight, do not consume whole wheat, but soy flour and rice or sprouted wheat.

Very beneficial: Rye Crisps, Rice Crackers, Essene Bread, Ezekiel Bread (available in some naturist houses), Unrefined Rice Bread, Rye Bread, Soy Flour Bread, Millet Bread, Wheat Bread Sprouted. "DIABETIC" people should suspend these foods until they are free of diabetes.

Neutrals: Arab Bread, Unleavened Bread, High Protein Bread, Spelled Bread, Non-Germinated Wheat Bread, Whole Wheat Bread, Gluten Free Bread, Oat Bran Bread, Wheat Bran Bread, Pumpernickel.

"DIABETIC" people should suspend these foods until they are free of diabetes.

Not Recommended: Breads or Meals of White or Yellow Corn Flour of Any Type.

GRAINS AND PASTA (noodles).

You benefit from rice instead of pasta, although you can eat semolina or spinach noodles once a week.

Substitute rye and oats for corn and wheat. Only eat bran and wheat germ once a week.

Very Beneficial: Basmatí Rice, White Rice, Indian Rice, Unrefined Rice, Rice Flour, Oat Rice, Rye Rice, Sprouted Wheat Rice.

"DIABETIC" people should suspend these foods until they are free of diabetes.

Neutrals: Couscous, Rice Pasta, Spinach Pasta, Semolina Pasta, Flour Gluten, Barley Pasta, Spelled Noodles, Graham Noodles, Bulgur Wheat Pasta, Wheat Noodles, Whole Wheat Noodles, Quinoa. "DIABETIC" people should suspend these foods until they are free of diabetes.

Not Recommended: Soba Noodles, Buckwheat Porridge, Artichoke Pasta, Corn-based Pasta, Sesame Paste (tahini).

VEGETABLES.

Avoid corn (jojoto, elote) and corn-based products.

Very Beneficial: Garlic, Celery, Sweet Potato (very little), Eggplant, Broccoli, Alfalfa Sprout, Cauliflower, Parsnip (white carrot), Dandelion, Mustard Leaves, Beet Leaves, Ginger, Carrot Juice (very little), Turnips, Potatoes (sweet potatoes, little), Parsnip, Cucumbers, Parsley, Green Cabbage, Tempeh (fermented soybeans), Tofu (tofu), Yam.

Neutral: Olives without Vinegar (green or black), Chard, Chicory, Agar (little), Caraway, Seaweed, Peas (peas), Pumpkin, Watercress, Green Cabbage, Bamboo Shoots, Zucchini, Chestnut (little), Onion of All Kinds, Kohlrabi, Chinese Cabbage, Brussels Sprouts, Coriander, Coriander, Shallots, Endives, Scallion, Endive, Asparagus, Spinach, Mushrooms, Fennel, Senna Leaves, Mushroom Enoki, Lettuce, Potato (little), Red Potato (little), Perifolio, Leek, Okra, Horseradish, Radicheta, Brussels Sprouts, Chinese Cabbage, Red Cabbage, White Cabbage, Arugula, Tomato without Shell, Cassava (VERY LITTLE), Carrot (little).

Not Recommended: Acacia (gum arabic), Avocado, Chili Peppers, Artichoke, Thistle, Chili, Shiitake Mushroom, Yellow Corn, White Corn, Chinese Ocumo, Products based on Aloe (zabila), Paprika, Radish, Rhubarb, Topinambur.

FRUITS.

Use the most alkaline ones like **grapes, plums, strawberries** to balance the acid-generating grains in your muscle tissue. **Avoid tropical fruits like orange, banana (cambur)** (there is also potassium in apricots (apricots), figs, and certain melons). **Pineapple is very beneficial.**

Very Beneficial: Blueberries (mirtillos), Cherries in General, Plums in General, Wild Currant, Dried Figs and Fresh Figs (WITHOUT SUGAR, less prickly pear),

Kiwi, Lime, Lemons, Pineapple (little), Grapefruit (grapefruit), Grape of any type (NO, AS LONG AS IT IS DIABETIC).

Neutral: Chinese Plum, Cocoa, Coconut (little), Damascus (apricot), Dates, Peach, Raspberry, strawberry, Soursop, Pineapple Juice (very little), Milky (papaya, little), Litchi, Mamón, Apple, Cantaloupe de all kinds (little), Peach, Blackberries, Chinese Orange, Nectarine (little), Parchita (little), watermelon (very little), Pears in General, Banana Parboiled (little), Prunas, Quinotos, Sauco, Zarzamora.

Not Recommended: Avocado, Bananas, Cambur, Persimmon or Kaki, Carambola, Granada, Guava, Fig of Tuna, Mangoes, Tangerine, Quinces, Oranges in General, Raisins, Pear Raft, Rhubarb.

JUICES AND LIQUIDS.

Drink a glass of warm water and the freshly squeezed juice of half a lemon every morning to clear the mucus and aid in evacuation. Then have a glass of diluted grapefruit juice. Choose alkaline fruit juices like **cranberry.**

Very Beneficial: Celery Juice, Cranberry Juice, Cherry Juice, Milky Juice (little), Cabbage Juice.

Neutrals: Coconut juice (little) Apple Cider, Plum Juice, Damascus Juice, Apple Juice, Cucumber Juice, Grapefruit Juice.

Not Advisable: Orange Juice, Guava Juice, Tangerine.

SPICES.

Table salt should be replaced by seaweed or seasoned sea salt from those sold in super markets, there are them for salads (Italian type), for seafood and for meats (sea salt should be moderate the amount of consumption, about all hypertensive). The dressing made with soy is very good and also makes a delicious soup or sauces. Avoid peppers **and vinegars** because they are acidic, use lemon juice with oil and herbs to dress salads and vegetables, and use garlic **a lot.**

Very Beneficial: Soy Dressing (natural), Garlic, Curry, Parsley, Ginger Root, Horseradish.

Neutral: Agar (seaweed jelly), Savory, Basil, Vinegar-free Capers , Caraway, Sea and Red Algae, Carob, Arrowroot, Saffron, Stevia Sugar (little), Bergamot, Cinnamon, Cocoa Powder, Cardamom, Chives, Cloves Spices, Coriander, Cumin, Cream of Tartar, Coriander, Turmeric, Chocolate without sugar , Dill, Tarragon, Wintergreen, Bay Leaf, Bay leaf, Yeast (little), Marjoram, Mint, Spearmint, Mustard Powder, Mustard without Vinegar , Nutmeg, Oregano, Paprika, Chervil, Paprika, Licorice Root, Rosemary, Sea Salt, Soy Sauce (NATURAL), Sage, Tamarind, Thyme, Cat's Claw.

Not Recommended: Chili Peppers, Vinegar Capers, Corn Starch (Cornstarch), Anise, Refined Sugar, Almond Extract (essence), Fructose, Pure Gelatin, Glucose, Corn Syrup, Maple Syrup, Junípero, Sugar Cane Syrup, Barley Malt, Honey, White or Black Pepper, Cayenne Pepper, Peppercorns, English Pepper, Black Pepper, Cider Vinegar, Vanilla, Wine Vinegar.

CONDIMENTS.

Do not eat seasonings in vinegar, excess salt and ketchup.

Very Beneficial: None.

Neutrals: Mayonnaise (without vinegar), Mustard without vinegar, Tomato Paste (homemade without vinegar).

Not Recommended: Pickles, Dill, Pickled Sweets, Kosher, Ketchup (tomato sauce, for the vinegar).

HERBAL INFUSIONS.

They should take herbal teas to boost the immune system and develop protection against cardiovascular disease and cancer.

Very Beneficial: Alfalfa, Burdock, Chamomile, Green Tea and Echinacea (excellent immune system stimulants), Marjoleto and Palo Dulce (for cardiovascular health), Dandelion, Burdock Root and

Strawberry Leaves (for iron absorption), Rose Hips, Ginseng, Ginger, Parsley.

Neutrals: White Birch, Alsine, Cayenne, White Oak Bark, Dong Quai, St. John's Wort, Catnip, Raspberry Leaf, Horehound, Yarrow, Mulberry, North American Elm, Mint, Sage, Elderberry, Thyme, Valerian, Verbena, Sarsaparilla.

Not Recommended: Fenugreek, Aloe (zabila), Corn Beard, Shepherd's Bag, Candlemas, Skullcap, Horse's Claw, Gentian, Hops, Rhubarb, Sen, Linden, Black Tea, Red Clover.

DRINKS (stimulants).

Very Beneficial: Ozonized Water. A Cup or Two of Green Tea per day Increases Gastric Acid Production and has the same enzymes as soybeans.

Neutral: Mineral Water, Lemon Water (water, little lemon), Seltz Water (carbonated water), Beer with little alcohol content (little), White Wine (no sugar and little), Red Wine (no sugar and little), (Wines, except the Hypertensive).

Not Advisable: Soft Drinks of Any Kind, Malt, Distilled Liquors, Black Tea (decaffeinated or common), Zabila Tea (aloe).

SUPPLEMENTS FOR TYPE AB.

They serve to strengthen the nervous system, provide antioxidants to fight cancer, and invigorate the heart.

Vitamin C: To protect against stomach cancer in doses less than 1 gr. since older ones can affect the stomach. It is suggested 2 to 3 capsules of 250 mg per day obtained from rose **hips** so that it does not cause digestive disorders. **Pineapple, broccoli, cherries, strawberries, lemon, and grapefruit** are rich in vitamin **C**.

Zinc: With caution, about 3 mg / day protects children from infections, especially from the ears, but higher long-term doses impair the immune system and interfere with the absorption of other minerals.

Take them under medical supervision. **There is zinc in recommended meats (especially dark turkey meat), eggs, and legumes.**

Selenium: It acts as a component of the body's antioxidant defenses. Check with your doctor.

Herbs and Phytochemicals for type AB.

Marjoleto (Crataegus oxyacantha): It is an antioxidant, increases the elasticity of the arteries and strengthens the heart muscle, reduces arterial hypertension and dissolves arterial plaques. It is sold in extracts and tinctures.

Immunity Enhancing Herbs: Echinacea (Echinacea Purpurea) prevents viral and infectious conditions

and ensures control of the immune system against cancer (liquid or tablets). Huang-ki (Astragalus membranaceous) as an immunizing tonic, but not readily available. The sugars in these two herbs act as mitogens by stimulating the production of white blood cells.

Soothing herbs: Chamomile, valerian root, infused.

Quercithin: Bioflavonoid found in yellow onion. It is a more powerful antioxidant than vitamin E and protects against cancer.

Mary thistle (Silybum marianum): An effective antioxidant that reaches high concentrations in the liver and bile ducts, indicated in those with a history of liver, pancreatic or gallbladder diseases. Also for patients treated with chemotherapy.

Bromeliad (pineapple enzyme): It has a moderate capacity to break down protein, contributing to its absorption.

FOODS THAT DEGENERATE.

- **Red meat: Poorly digested, it is stored as fat.**
- **Beans: Inhibit insulin efficiency causing hypoglycemia.**
- **Beans-beans: Inhibit insulin efficiency, cause hypoglycemia.**
- **Sesame seeds: They cause hypoglycemia:**
- **Wheat: Slows metabolism inefficient use of calories and also inhibits insulin efficiency.**

FOODS THAT REGENERATE.

- **Tofu: Promotes metabolic efficiency.**
- **Fish: They promote metabolic efficiency.**
- **Dairy: They improve insulin production.**
- **Vegetables: They improve metabolic efficiency.**
- **Seaweed: Improves insulin production.**
- **Pineapple: Facilitates digestion and stimulates bowel movements.**

OTHER RECOMMENDATIONS...

- **Healthy Longevity Book... How to Live 100 Years Appearing Much Less.**

- **The Cookbook... Personalized According to your Blood Group.**

- **Certified Courses for Professionals and Aspiring Therapists.**

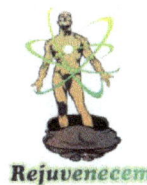

The House of Children Foundation...
We recommend the "BOOK TO HEALTHY LONGEVITY GROUP A DIABETIC".
The goal... Live 100 years Appearing much less... Because if you can... **Bring:**

➤ How to eat and Rejuvenate according to your Blood Group.

➤ Special Exercises to Increase Health.

➤ Golden Tips that will make you lead a Much Better Life.

➤ How to eat after 45.

➤ How to Regenerate Metabolism.

➤ How to clean the liver, bile ducts, colon and kidneys.

➤ Alkalinity Life - Acids Death.

➤ How Emotional Conflicts Kill.

➤ Why We Age and How to Rejuvenate (2,023)...

➤ Local and Systemic Mushroom Cleaning

➤ 9 Foods to Have More Intense Intimate Relationships.

➤ The 12 Best Nutrients for Life Extension.

THE KITCHEN RECIPE FOR DIABETIC GROUP A...

It is personalized according to your blood group, where you can prepare delicacies that will rejuvenate you and in a simple way.... Bring:

➤ How to Prepare the Best Sauces.

➤ How to Prepare the Best Mayonnaise.

➤ Preparation of Smoked Bones at home.

➤ Prepare the best Chimichurri or Guasacaca that you have ever eaten.

➤ Italian Sea Salt, For Salads, Meats, Seafood, Fish and Poultry.

➤ Broths for: Meat, Seafood, Chicken, Chicken, Fish.

➤ Unrivaled Starters, Salads, Soups, Creams and Main Dishes.

➤ Yyyy of course the best Christmas dishes.

And remember that your Blessing will Help Many Needy here at La Casa De DIOS Foundation and where we will be praying for your seed to be paid in health for you and you're Family.

The Cookbook will find it at this link. www.fundaciondeterapeutas.com

COURSES.

✚ Certified Courses for Professionals and Aspiring Therapists.

Sai-Medic Institute for Scientific Research.
Attacking the Cause. Effects Disappear.
Center for Alternatives
Scientific Health Research.

Rejuveneceme

With more than 45 years of experience in hundreds of thousands of patients and using the latest advances in science, we will indicate you with simple, but powerful recommendations, how to treat the problems that afflict humanity in such a fast and palpable way, that you will believe. Find out why we get sick and age. How to quickly rejuvenate and heal...

Ownership of the Course Certified by the Institute will be delivered.

Professional Courses.

COURSE Chosen.

1- Neuro Advanced Acupuncture. Energy Systems.

2- Food to have more intense relationships.

3- How to Regenerate According to the Blood Group.

4- How to Rejuvenate.

5- Cancer If Cured.

6- Obesity ... Lose Weight Immediately.

7- How to cure type 2 diabetes in a short time.

"May GOD be our Strength"

CURRICULUM VITAE

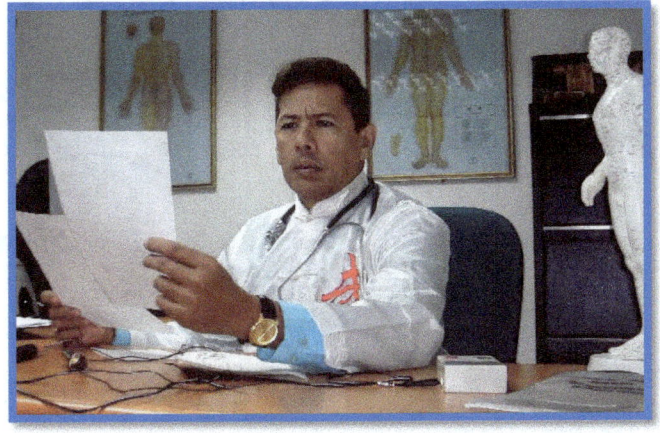

Name: M. A Ramoni

Web: fundaciondeterapeutas.com

Professional Studies:

➤ ENAHO (National School of Acupuncture and Homeopathy). Years 1983 to 1989.

➤ Studies at the Venezuelan School of Psychotronic Society. 1989 Caracas Venezuela.

➤ Studies of the Food Yin Yang Macrobiotic knowledge of Dr. Sakurazawa Nyoiti of Japanese origin, through Professor Omar Viera.

➤ Korean Acupuncture (Koryo Sooji Chim Acupuncture Mano koryo) from Master Dr. Yoo Tae W received with a Three Level program at the National School of Acupuncture and Homeopathy through Dr. Omar Viera.

➤ Studies of Dr. José Luís Padilla Corral, director of the School of MT Ch. "Neijing" Spain.

➤ Regression hypnosis INME Institute (Experimental Meta-gnomic Institute).

➤ Didactic Homeosineatry. From the Bathem Bathen school.

➤ Iridology. International Federation of Iris Diagnosis. From the Federation of Dr. Omar Viera.

➤ Maxilo-Facial anti-wrinkle treatment through the dermatron and electo-acupuncture. 2009 (I continue).

➤ Food According to the Blood Group. Research researcher James and Peter D'adamo. 2008. (I continue).

➤ Rejuvenation through the lengthening of the telomeres. 2010 (I continue).

➤ Alkalinity and acidity of cells in the development of diseases. 2010 (I continue).

➤ Master in Energy Systems.

- Master in Anesthesia by Electro Acupuncture.

- Master in Pain Therapies.

- Master in Iridology (Diagnosis by Iris).

- Neuropsychology. The New Medicine of the Future. Dr Hamer Germany.

JOBS:

- President and founder of the Scientific Research Institute of Alternative Health Medicines SAID-MEDIC.

- Director of the Said-Medic La Maracaya Medical Center clinic from 1988 to 1992.

- Director of the Said-Medic Lourdes Medical Center clinic from 1993 to 1995.

- Director of the Said-Medic Medical Center clinic Dungeon from the year 1996 to the year 2,000.

- Professor in courses for Doctors and Para-Doctors in Homeopathy - Acupuncture 1st Level - 2nd Level - 3rd Level and Energy Systems.

➤ Director of the Las Acacias Said-Medic Medical Center clinic from the year 2010 to the year 2012.

➤ Director of the Said-Medic Palmarito Medical Center clinic from year 2013 to year 2017.

➤ Director of the Said-Medic Street Páez Medical Center clinic from 2.017 to 2.023.

➤ Professor, Lecturer, International Bioenergetics Seminary - Neuro Acupuncture - Food according to the Blood Group - Why we age and how to rejuvenate - Main diseases, Neuro Psychology, among others.

WRITER OF MEDICINE BOOKS:

1- Rejuvenate, lose weight, be strong and healthy.

2- Food According to Blood Group "O".

3- Blood Group Healthy Longevity Guide A.

4- Blood Group Healthy Longevity Guide A Diabetic.

5- Blood Group Healthy Longevity Guide AB.

6- Blood Group Healthy Longevity Guide Ab Diabetic.

7- Blood Group Healthy Longevity Guide B.

8- Blood Group Healthy Longevity Guide B Diabetic.

9- Blood Group Healthy Longevity Guide O.

10- Blood Group Healthy Longevity Guide O Diabetic.

11- Food According to Blood Group "A"

12- Food According to Blood Group "B"

13- Food According to the Blood Group "AB"

14- Food According to the Diabetic Blood Group "O"

15- Food According to the Diabetic Blood Group "A"

16- Food According to the Diabetic Blood Group "B"

17- Food According to the Diabetic Blood Group "AB"

18- Blood Group **Cookery Recipe** "O".

19- Blood Group **Cookbook** "A"

20- Blood Group **Cookbook** "B"

21- Blood Group **Cookbook** "AB"

22- **Cooking Recipe** Group Diabetic Blood "O"

23- **Cooking Recipe** Group Diabetic Blood "A"

24- **Cooking Recipe** Diabetic Blood Group "B"

25- **Cooking Recipe** Diabetic Blood Group "AB"

26- Cancer if cured ... Educate, Alkalize and Balance.

27- Slimy Blood Syndrome ... The Cause of All Diseases.

28- How to Cure the Prostate.

29- Free yourself from Arthritis.

30- Farewell to Rheumatism.

31- Obesity ... Lose Weight Immediately and never Gain Fat again.

32- Alkalinity Life - Acidity Death.

33- Diabetes if Cured.

34- Say Goodbye to Hypertension.

35- Constipation ... Dark Future.

36- Convert your Pain into Well-being ... Legs, Lumbago, Sciatica, Spine and Cervical, among others.

37- Regenerate yourself from ACV

38- How to Eliminate Kidney and Gallstones.

39- Liver, Bile Duct, Gallbladder and colon cleansing

40- Cure Gastritis and Gastro Esophageal Reflux.

41- Say goodbye to asthma.

42- Because we grow old.

43- Tell me your Conflict ... And I will tell you that you suffer.

OTHER BOOKS:

1- CROSS POETRY. (Poetry, Updating).

2- 7 MINUTES. (Thriller, Updating).

PROFESSIONAL ASSOCIATIONS:

✚ Member of the WHO (World health organization number 0023 for Latin America, in alternative health medicines, through ENAHO).

✚ Member of the International Acupunture Association.

✚ College of Homeopaths and Natural Alternative Medicine Sciences.

✚ Venezuelan Federation of Natural Alternative Medicines N° 0024V as well as Member of the International Centers of Homeopathy and

Acupuncture of: CHCMANV N° CHV002-A - INCIHOVE N° 00020 AVA 051-V.

SPECIALTIES.

1- Diagnostic Specialist.

2- Cancer if cured.

3- Neuropathies.

4- Column.

5- Cervicals.

6- Some (pain) of any kind.

7- Type 2 and 3 diabetes If it is cured.

8- Type 1 diabetes (Mellitus) exponentially improves the quality of life.

9- Arthritis.

10-   Rheumatism.

11-   Obesity.

12-   Diseases without Cause Diagnosis.

13-   Migraine, Headache.

14-   Digestive System.

15-   ACV

16- Body, Mental and Dynamic Rejuvenation.

17- Asthma.

18- Allergies.

19- Lupus.

20- Emotional Conflicts.

21- Traumas.

22- Renal Deficiency.

23- Neurological Senile dementia, Parkinson's, Alzheimer's, Huntington.

24- Seizures.

25- Hypertension ... Among many others.

"If we eliminate the cause ... the effects are eliminated."

"The Course that Rules Nature ...

It is the Artistic Expression of *GOD*."

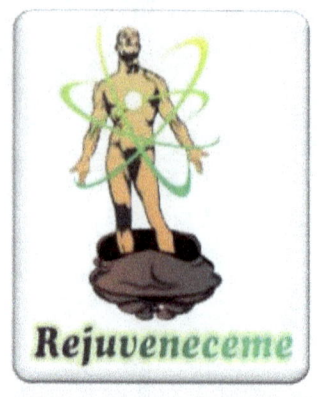

Now, reread one by one the important topics that you will find in the Healthy Longevity Guide, in relation to the new culture of rejuvenation - healing and get rid of once and forever, that damaged state that so much hinders a body healthy.

www.fundaciondeterapeutas.com   2.023.

DEDICATION...

I want to dedicate this and all the good things I have done in this world to the one who deserves it the most and that is my Heavenly Father.

Jehovah of Hosts...

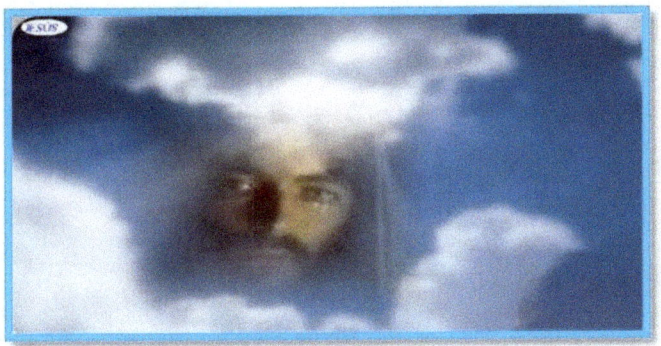

Thank you, I love you very much and... In the name of **GOD** ...I wish you the best...

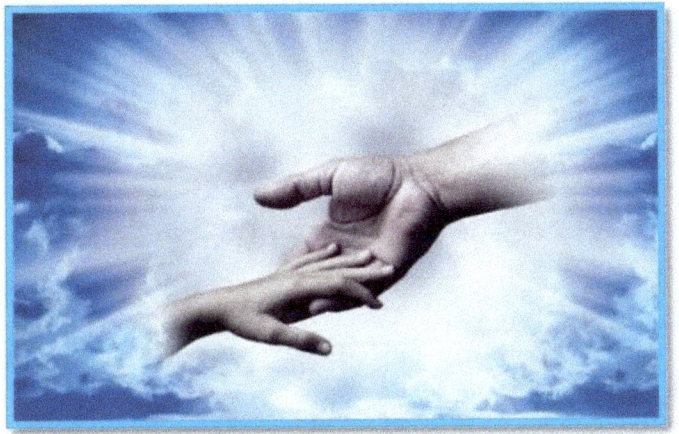

So... Never forget, that when science says... I can't anymore... **GOD** says... I start...

www.ingramcontent.com/pod-product-compliance
Lightning Source LLC
Chambersburg PA
CBHW072305170526
45158CB00003BA/1191